Legal & Disclaimer

Contents

Introduction

I congratulate you on downloading this book and hope to pass along information to you that will help you in your quest for a flat belly. If you have been trying to lose belly fat and have not been able to accomplish it, this book is for you. If you have never tried to find a program to help you lose belly fat, this book is for you. You have come to the right place. Getting rid of belly fat can be simple or difficult depending on how you look at what you have to do to eliminate the belly fat. The important thing is to sum up the goddess within by feeling confident with yourself when you have lost the fat from your belly.

I want you to know that you can eliminate your belly fat. This book looks at the emotional and physical changes that you will go through while on this 30 day exercise plan. This book will help you step back and see the big picture so that you can put in motion the exercises and diet plan and carry on living your life. You do not want belly fat to consume your life, you have better things to do.

You are going to have to change some of your daily routines in order to eliminate belly fat, but these exercises are not very intrusive in your day. You are going to have to change your diet a bit, but don't worry. I am not telling you to eliminate everything that you eat, and you will not necessarily have to give up the comfort food that you love. You will have to change the way in which you eat the things that you are eating. You will also have to make some other minor changes. These changes will be worth it because at the end of 30-Days you will have a flatter stomach.

Having a flatter belly will make you look and feel much better. When you look in the mirror you will be proud of the body that you see. The main focus is what you do to get a flatter belly. The entire process is going to make you feel better, look better, and give you better health. The goddess within you is awaiting to come forth. Taking care of yourself will help with your longevity and improve your health and immune system.

You have taken the first step in getting a flatter belly by buying this book. I am not asking you to buy any cream, solution, or pill of any kind, because you do not need one. This is an overall exercise and health plan that you will be able to carry with you for the rest of your life. Try to get as much support as you can from your friends and family as well. Support helps in the overall success of this plan and reaching the goal of a flatter belly.

Rest assure that this is a plan you can incorporate into your life. Incorporate them as part of your lifestyle and you will begin to experience positive changes. You will have more control over these exercises and eating habits. When you have control, you get more done and feel good about the situation at hand. It is important that you read and reread this book so you have full confidence in what you are doing. This will help you succeed in your battle against belly flat.

I have all the confidence in you that you can succeed with this plan. If you put in the effort to make this plan work, you will be so happy with your body's transformation. Thirty days from now you will hold your head higher because your stomach is firmer, making you feel youthful and more confident. So let's take a look at how to flatten your belly in 30 days.

Grab Free Books Here

From time to time, I would highlight to my readers some interesting books which I found on Kindle. Subscribe to our newsletter to receive free bestselling kindle books recommendation delivered to your inbox daily. You can subscribe to our newsletter by clicking on the link below:

http://giveaway.kindleheaven.com/index.php/kindle-free-book/

It is 100% free and there will not be a single spam email. Just pure sharing of good books with my readers.

Please also like our facebook page below to get recommendation on good books to read for the day.

https://www.facebook.com/Kindle-Heaven-1651266215134798

Follow us on Twitter to get tweets on worthwhile books

https://twitter.com/KindleHeaven

Chapter 1: Anatomy of A Flat Belly

Understand what makes your belly fat and your 30 day journey will be much easier. If you avoid the things that put fat on your belly then you can get a flat belly and maintain it. First, it is important to consult your doctor before attempting any type of diet. Everyone has different dietary needs and body composition. If you have health issues of any kind you want to consult your doctor about the details of your diet and exercise. Make sure your diet and exercise fit your particular body.

So what puts fat on the belly? The numbers can vary, but most women should eat about 1200 to 1500 calories a day. Of course, the number of calories each woman needs may vary depending on what a woman does. It would be great idea to consult a nutritionist who can tell you the proper calorie intake you need depending on your individual lifestyle. On average eating 1200 to 1500 calories of food a day is plenty to be healthy. Now, if a woman eats day after day, say 1800 or more calories every day, then she will start to gain weight. This can lead to belly fat build up. If you eat more than 1200 calories for one day and then go back to eating 1200 to 1500 calories you won't gain weight. It is the repetition of overeating that causes the fat to build up on different parts of your body. Also, it is important to know that a woman can't just eat 1200 calories of any kind to prevent belly fat. She has to eat certain types of food that will help reduce and maintain a flat stomach.

Lack of activity can cause a woman's body to gain belly fat. Your body naturally burns at least 1200 calories per day in its resting state. It is important for a woman to stay active and perform activities that raise her heartbeat and makes her sweat. However, the chosen sport must be fun and cannot be stressful. Less stress keeps the frown and wrinkles away from the goddess within.

Also, drink lots of water. Water is a carrier. The purpose of drinking water is to carry the nutrients of the food you have eaten all throughout your body, as well as to take the waste out every day. If you do not drink enough water, your body will build up waste and you can easily gain belly fat this way. It is absolutely important to drink enough water everyday to maintain a flat belly. The amount of water you need to drink will be in the coming chapters.

You must rest and relax everyday to help maintain a flat belly. What happens when you try to starve yourself too much in one day? Your body will hoard the calories you have and you will put on weight. Your belly can be the first place you gain weight. Your body will always fight to give you enough nutrients to survive. So resting at night is imperative for a flat belly. Relaxing after meals and little breaks mid morning and mid afternoon will help to keep away belly fat.

How you breathe and keep stress to a minimum can make or break your belly fat. When you breathe properly, and carry yourself in a way that uses your stomach muscles then you are helping to keep belly fat away.

These are some of the small details that can make a lot of difference. As you age you will find that you gain belly fat more easily. It does not have to be that way. You just have to follow a few simple rules to maintain a flat belly.

Chapter 2: Preparing Your Exercise Plan

You want to mentally and physically prepare yourself for your thirty day exercise plan. When it is time to start your exercise plan you want to have everything ready. The combination of eating well, sleeping, activity, and relaxing all plays a role in reducing belly fat and maintaining a flat belly. You want to make your belly fat reduction experience as easy as possible. Everything may seem a bit instructional and boring at first, but you have to remember that the goal is to have a flat belly, so some control is necessary at first. You will have plenty of time to relax later. First, you want to pick a comfortable place in your house to do your exercises. Choose a location where you are free to move around and have enough space for you to lie on the floor. Buy yourself a large towel, sheet, or blanket to place on the floor. You want to buy something specifically for your exercise. You may also need a mirror so you can see the progress of your workout better. Make sure there is plenty of room to prevent injury by mistake. Try to find a place in your house where you will not be interrupted. If you can exercise alone, it is best. If you have a supportive group of friends that will help you through your weight loss and want to do the exercises too, this is okay. Just make sure that the exercise time is positive and productive.

You will also need to prepare sufficient drinking water. You will need about three to four liters of water a day. It is recommended that you drink this amount daily. Two 1.5 liter tall thin bottles with an additional one liter bottle of water is good. Anytime you need to drink during these thirty days, use the water from these bottles. You want to see that the bottles are empty at the end of the day. This way you get an idea of how much water you drink. Where possible, buy a BHP free plastic bottle and a distiller as these two things are really good and healthy. You can also buy a gallon and just drink the gallon by the end of the day. Your entire drinking source will come from the three to four liters water. You will have to stop drinking other drinks for a little while, especially those high in calories, sugar, and artificial flavors.

Getting sufficient sleep is very important for your skin and beauty regeneration. Try to get up at the same time everyday. Just set your alarm accordingly and you will start the rhythm. Going to bed early is the hardest part sometimes. You need at least eight hours of sleep, six at the very least. It is important to realize that certain things can wait until tomorrow and they should. You need your sleep for proper weight loss and overall health.

It is important that you set up your exercise routine to be a thirty minute block of time. Get your workout done first thing in the morning. Evenings are for your rest and relaxation. For a nice flat stomach you want to try to workout anywhere from the time you get-up till before 6:00. You do not want to work out on an empty stomach. If you eat in the morning, then let your food digest a bit while you brush your teeth, or any other tasks you can do while waiting. About twenty five to thirty minutes after you eat, start stretching and getting yourself warmed up to do the exercises.

Consistency is the key to success. While a little variation is fun, losing the belly fat requires determination and discipline. So just to recap you will need to prepare for your belly flat exercises by stocking three to four liters of water in advance on your kitchen counter every day. Then pick your designated area and have a clean towel or blanket on standby. Finally, you will want to set your wake-up and sleeping times. Before we take a look at the exercises, let's take a look at the food to eat while on the diet plan.

Chapter 3: Foods to Eat While on the 30 Day Belly Flat Plan

I wish I could tell you that you could eat donuts for thirty days and do the belly flat exercises and you would still have a flat belly, but this can never happen. It is very important that you eat the right food when you are on your belly fat crusade. The good news is you will be able to eat whatever you want if you just follow a couple of simple rules.

If you eat foods that block up your system, then your belly will continue to grow fat. If you feed your body the right kinds of foods most of the time, you can keep belly fat to a minimum. Always remember to eat food in small portions. Three meals a day are important and get some healthy snacks in between. This helps increase your metabolism.

The main focus of any healthy body is to eat a nice balance of vegetables, fruits, whole grains, protein, and some treats. There are so many foods that fall under this category that you will never be bored eating this way.

If you have been eating foods that are processed or boxed then you may need a little time to adjust. You want to stay away from processed foods of any kind. This is crucial to reduce belly fat. Eat more whole foods. Eating whole foods gets your system working on a cycle of nourishing yourself and then eliminating what you don't need on a daily basis.

Foods you can eat within the 1200-1500 calories are wonderful foods like chicken, fish, and beans. You can have red meat about once a week. If you want a sandwich, make it whole grain with veggies. Only eat chips once a week and just one serving size. Nuts are also a great source of protein. Coconut is great for flavoring foods or even as snack. Bananas make excellent fillers. The choice is yours with vegetables. You can have them for lunch and for dinner. Salads are excellent for either meal, but make sure you have protein like a couple ounces of chicken or fish.

It is important that you go to the produce isle of your grocery store and start finding out vegetables you like. You will be eating two servings a day if not more, one serving at lunch, and one serving at dinner. You can also have the vegetable medleys from the frozen food isle as well. Olive oil is a great protein and flavor for vegetables and salads. Garlic and onion will flavor almost anything you cook. During the thirty days, before you eat anything, ask yourself does this fall under the category of vegetable, fruit, protein, whole grain, nut or bean. If it does not, move on until you find those foods that fit into the category.

Chapter 4: Seven Flat Belly Exercises to Start Today

The key to the belly fat exercises is that you must like them. When you are doing exercises that you like, you are more apt to keep doing those exercises. Here are some of the main belly fat reduction exercises. Breathe in and out through all these exercises. A nice steady breathe is important for weight loss. Be conscious of your breath throughout all exercises.

Exercise One

Lay on the floor on your back on top of a sheet, towel, or blanket. Press your shoulders and buttocks onto the floor. Place your hands by your sides. Push your heels onto the floor. Next stretch your right arm out to your side. Next bring the knee of your right leg halfway up to your chest so it is parallel to your pelvis and then cross your knee over your body to your left side and touch the floor with your knee. If you can't touch the floor yet just go as far as you can go. Then bring your knee back across your body and put it back down so you are flat again. Do this ten times. Work up to twenty repetitions. Next, stretch your left arm out and lift your left leg and knee, and cross over your body. Repeat on this side ten times at first and then work up to twenty. Just do twenty per day for five to six days a week.

Exercise Two

Lay down on the floor and prop your knees up with your feet flat on the floor and your buttocks and back flat on the floor. Your knees will be bent pointing to the ceiling. Clasp your hands behind your back with elbows out to the side. Now pull yourself up with your stomach and touch your forehead to your knees. It is similar to the regular sit-up, but you want to make sure you follow through by touching nose to knees. You also want to make sure that your back curls off the floor and you keep your stomach pressed to the floor from the top. That may sound weird but you can do it. You don't want your stomach flopping all over the place. It should be one fluid motion and then slowly lower yourself back to the ground. Do ten repetitions on the first day and slowly work your way up to twenty. This may seem like a sit-up and it is very close. They both use and strengthen your stomach very well.

Exercise Three

Lay on your back flat on the floor, and spread your legs so they make a V. Place your feet flat on the floor. You will be supporting yourself with your shoulders and your feet flat on the floor. The point of this exercise is to lift your buttocks off the floor and squeeze your entire mid section. You will be supporting yourself with the tip of your shoulders and your feet flat on the ground and your legs. You will raise your buttocks and squeeze your mid section and then lower your back to the ground. Repeat this ten times the first day and then work up to twenty times. Do twenty a day. Give yourself a break no more than two days a week.

Exercise Four

Stand with your legs spread apart and your hands up in the air so you create an X with your body. Reach down with your right hand and touch your left foot and come back up. Then reach down with your left and touch your right foot. As you are going down to touch your foot keep your hand close to your body, by running your hand down your body smoothly until you get to your feet. Repeat this ten times the first day and twenty times all other days.

Exercise Five

Again stand with your legs apart. With your left hand on your hip raise your right arm above your head and lean over to your left side. It might help to look in the mirror when you are doing this exercise. Only go so far so that you get a nice stretch in your side. Slightly bounce back and forth as your arm is over on the side and count ten the first day then twenty the next day and for all following days.

Exercise Six

Lay flat on your back on the floor and put your hands behind your head with your elbows out. Lift your right leg and bring your knee up to your chest towards your left elbow and then put your leg back down. Now lift your left leg and bring your knee into your chest towards your right elbow and then put your foot back down. Do ten repetitions back and forth from one leg to the next. Work up to twenty repetitions a day.

Final Exercise

After you complete these floor exercises you want to pick an activity that raises your heartbeat for at least fifteen minutes of continuous motion. Running and dancing are the two simplest ways to keep your heartbeat up. The point of this exercise is to move all your body parts, raise your heartbeat and start to sweat. Always pay attention to your breathing. You can breathe in through your nose and out through your mouth if you want. Pick one activity and stick to it, whether it is swimming soccer or basketball. Remember you need to perform 20 minutes of activity at least five days a week. Getting frequent exercise also stimulates the production of adiponectin and leptin that will help your body burn even more fat.

Chapter 5: Emotional and Physical Changes to Expect

Changing the way you eat, exercise, and live your daily life is excellent, but it can be a little difficult because of the emotional and physical changes that you will go through. Everyday is a new day and poses a new challenge for getting through the diet experience. The main point of this book is to get you on a simple path of health that will work for you.

You may lose the drive to do your exercises every morning. You may even not feel like doing these exercises at all. This can be quite normal, but at first you might have to push yourself to do things you do not want to. If you push yourself you will start to see the results you desire. If you can't overcome your emotions, you may want to quit, but don't. You will be so happy when you push through. Push yourself for 21 straight days and it will become a habit in no time.

You will run into moments where you don't think your body is changing. You may run into moments where you don't think anything is happening, don't worry. This is normal, just keep doing the exercises. The reality is that you have to do something for at least four weeks to start seeing successful results. Everyone will start at a different level, and everyone will be at a different place at the end of thirty days. If you stick with the plan, you will see the light at the end of the tunnel.

Your muscles may hurt at first until you have strengthened them enough. Muscles that haven't been used in a while usually ache. You are looking to have control over your muscles instead of being so relaxed in your body. Muscles have to be stretched and moved in all directions and used in order to strengthen them and keep them strong. You will start to feel the difference in your stomach when you can hold it in with comfort. The more you work your stomach muscles the easier it will be to carry yourself in a good way.

Be conscious of how you carry yourself by looking in the mirror. Walk towards the mirror and see what you look like when you are walking. It is an interesting lesson to see how you look to the world. Looking in the mirror and forming a positive opinion of yourself is good. It gives you positive reinforcement about your looks. Make sure whoever it is with you is being true to you and your feelings.

When you start to see some results, you are going to start feeling good. When this happens, you may get carried away and break your pattern. Just keep steady with all that you are doing and enjoy your success. Everyday is a day to feel good about yourself and how you are living your life. Try not to crash and burn and over celebrate. Sometimes people consider looking good as an end point, but it is a place of contentment and maintenance. You have to continue to do your exercises and eat well to have a flat belly. The sad thing is muscles have no memory so if you don't use them they will atrophy and lose their strength. You won't want that to happen, because feeling and looking good will make you want to continue your exercise plan.

You may think that doing more activity and repetitions is going to help, but be very careful with this. You can easily get bored and quit. The reason to do less rather than more is to help you maintain this plan over the long run. This way you won't have to think about having to diet and exercise ever again, because you just live a healthy lifestyle that makes you feel good.

Physical changes, lack of progress, lack of desire, over-celebrating, doing more than you should, having a positive and realistic view of how you look to the world are all physical and emotional changes you will experience on the 30 day belly flat program. These changes can be challenging for you, but you can cope. Master the belly flat program so that you will eventually just be on the maintenance plan for your strength and good health.

You may notice your weight either go up a little, down, and sometimes nowhere at all. This is normal. You want to see where you are at the end of the week. You can step on the scale at the beginning of the week and watch the numbers of the scale every day for the first seven days, but take it with a grain of salt. Don't panic too much if the weight fluctuates. Just stick to the plan and you will eventually reach your goal. If you get too intimidated by the scale, just follow the plan and weigh yourself at the end of 30 days if you like.

Chapter 6: The ONE Secret That Guarantees Success With The Program

It is nice to know that you will have a flatter belly when you put in the time to exercise and eat right, but sometimes sheer discipline is not enough. It is important to focus on something else while waiting for your stomach to flatten. You want to pick a reward for yourself every week for following the plan. You want to pick a reward that means a lot to you, something that will inspire you if you get emotionally low. By rewarding yourself you will be able to keep yourself on this exercise plan.

Pick just one reward a week. Some examples would be like a cup of ice cream or a candy bar. If you eat one treat like this it will not stop the overall weight loss in your belly. You can also choose a reward that is more stimulating like a new phone or a new shirt. Think about what you would like and set your sight on buying this treat. You can only have the rewards if you honestly put forth the effort of eating well and doing your exercises at least five days a week.

Other things you can do to reward yourself is to take care of your body. Oils and lotions that keep your skin moisturized will help in the long run. You want to keep your hair well-groomed at all time. Your finger nails and toe nails need to be trimmed. Looking good is a reward in itself, but it helps to give yourself a little extra time to say thank you for your hard work. Looking good and staying strong can sometimes feel like hard work, but the reward far outweighs the effort. Eventually what seems like work just becomes the new normal. You will feel happy to do exercises once you see the result from doing them.

You may sometimes doubt why you have to take care of yourself at all. The ultimate reward is that eventually if you take care of your body, mind, and soul you can keep yourself out of the hospital. From eating well, exercising, and resting you are helping yourself as you age. You are also closing the window of opportunity for sickness to set in easily. Taking care of yourself can help you live a longer life, and a better life overall. When you take care of yourself, you will have the confidence to call upon the goddess within and just be her.

So remember it is of utmost importance to pick one reward for yourself and work towards giving it to yourself after the first seven days of your program. Then start another seven day cycle and give yourself the same reward or a different one. Never stop giving yourself that reward once a week as a token of appreciation for putting in the work to keep yourself healthy, happy and strong. Looking good takes effort but you can do it.

Chapter 7: How to Maintain a Flat Belly

I hope you have found the exercises in this book useful. I hope you have been doing them for some time now. After thirty days, your belly area should be flatter, and you should be looking better. You of course have to follow all the instructions in order to see real results. Sometimes it is helpful to write a journal about your experience, or even write a list of the tasks you have to do to succeed with the diet plan. Writing a list helps you remember all the details of the diet. You can also plug in the details to your Smartphone and include alarms for times as well. You can use your Smartphone or Iphone to play music and keep track of the time of your twenty minute heartbeat raising activity.

You may think ahhh, thirty days this is it and my belly is flat. A diet is not an end point it is the beginning of a way of life. You have to continue to do your exercises. You have to continue to eat well and your belly will get flatter and stronger. You will reach a point where your belly will be as flat as you want it to be. From this point on you will just be doing the exercises for maintenance. Please do not think you can stop your exercises all together. If you stop the exercises over time your belly can become flabby again. You do not want to waste all your effort by stopping your belly exercises. Continue to do them and eat well and you will preserve your good looking body, and maintain your health and overall wellbeing.

As far as eating goes, avoid foods that are not good for your health. It is no different than it has been while you are on your diet. You can have food that is fattening or sugary as your reward once a week, be it potato chips, cheesecake, or triple fudge Sunday. The main point is that you must eat in moderation and maintain a serving size within your 1200 to 1500 calories per day. Enjoy yourself. Fattening foods don't make people fat, it's the amount we eat that does.

Always keep your emotions in check when eating. Also, not eating on time can set your emotions off. If you don't eat and feed yourself properly, it can create bad moods which can lead to bad decisions. Always try to eat first and do what you have to do next. Many people, especially in America, do first and eat later and this causes the body to go into storage mode where the body holds on to the food you ate the last time. If your body does not believe you are going to feed it, it will store fat. Make sure you take control of your body as opposed of your body.

Please remember to never stop taking care of yourself. There is no cure all solutions to weight loss. You must put in the time and effort. You must deny yourself some things sometimes and then give yourself a little at other times. This is a more scientific approach to the matter. Treat the body right and it will give you back what you want: a strong and healthy appearance.

Special Bonus

To thank you for purchasing my guide, I have specifically prepared the bonus **"Hijacking The Holiday Weight Gain"** report for you. This report will show you how you can enjoy your holiday binge without putting on any weight.

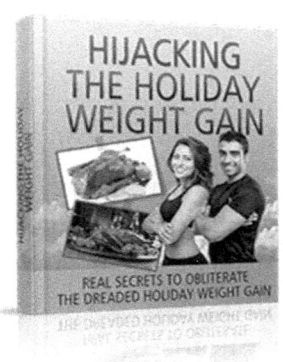

Inside this report, you will find:

1. Simple nutrition strategies to boost your metabolism during holidays

2. A full example of a holiday exercise routine

3. And many more….

To download this special bonus, simply visit this URL below:

http://giveaway.kindleheaven.com/index.php/holiday-diet/

….And put in both your name and email there so I know who to address and which email address to send the report to

Conclusion

The most important thing to do is to love yourself. You have to love all your flaws and all your advantages. Wanting a flatter belly is a good but taking care of yourself is more important. It is so easy to get caught up in all the great pleasures of food and laziness, or over work yourself for the concept of money and self sacrifice. You deserve to be happy. These are the things that the 30 Day belly flat plan is here to help you with.

Try to enjoy every step of the process. Seek out the energy of the program that moves you forward from day to day. When you feel good, everyone feels good around you. When you feel good about yourself, you want to do more and contribute more.

Find support wherever you can get it. Push through the hard times of the program no matter what. You may have tried other programs in the past and failed. Don't let the same mistake haunt you.

Keep following your bliss within the confines of the program. If you need to switch-up your twenty minute activity to something else, this is fine. The most important thing is to move continuously. You want to move your body all over to burn more fat. The stomach strengthening exercises are just as important, because they build your core and help create the definition in your stomach that you desire. Listening to music you love while working out makes it more enjoyable.

I can't stress enough the importance of the portion control of food. There are so many theories out there for weight loss, that people forget the good old fashion way that has worked for people for years. Just don't overeat. We overeat because it feels good, but then we feel bad when we are too fat. So if you just eat a regular portion, you will get to eat what you like, and not pack on the pounds. If you like something, save it for the next meal, or the next day. You don't have to eat everything in one sitting. There is always another meal.

I hope everything in this book speaks to you and helps you on your quest for a flat belly. I congratulate you if you have already started the exercises. Do whatever it takes to get yourself healthy. Thank you again for reading and I wish the best of luck, always!

-- Virginia Miller